Essential Oils:
Over 30 Warming Blends for Diffusers

The information herein is offered for informational purposes solely, and is universal as so. The presentation of the information is without contract or any type of guarantee assurance.

The trademarks that are used are without any consent, and the publication of the trademark is without permission or backing by the trademark owner. All trademarks and brands within this book are for clarifying purposes only and are the owned by the owners themselves, not affiliated with this document.

Table of content

Introduction

An essential oil is a intense liquid that is thick in consistency and contains aromatic compounds that are derived from plants. Commonly known as the oil of the plant, essential oils are an extract of the plant and as they are the purest form of the plant's fragrance.

These essential oils are pull out by distillation procedure and by use of steam while other methods include solvent extraction and even cold pressing. They are used for making cosmetics, perfumes, soaps and even for food flavoring. One of the most popular uses of essential oils that became very common is adding fragrances to domestic cleaning products as these oils are natural and contain very strong fumes.

If we go back in history, we will see that essential oils were used in medicine by ancient people. There were medical practitioners who made use of these essential oils to treat skin problems and other ailments. There have also been evidences where essential oils were used to treat cancer patients that show how beneficial they have been in the past too.

Interest in essential oils has revived in the present too and with aromatherapy gaining popularity among the masses, people are now turning towards essential oils and trying to understand how they can use them for improving their quality of life. It is necessary to know that these essential oils are volatile aroma compounds and they have curative effects that help people deal with their mental as well as physical problems.

When used in a diffuser, these essential oils can be used for various purposes from keeping the air fresh and scented to using it for creating warming blends for winter that help people suffering from various ailments. With help of diffusers, one can discover the transformative and aromatic power of essential oils that help to stay calm and healthy.

Chapter 01: Holiday Diffuser Blends for Winter

During winter many people face problems like wheezing or bad cold and congestions but with help of essential oils, they can alleviate their problems and make sure they enjoy better health quality. All they need to understand is which diffuser blends of essential oils they should use for winter that keep their ailments in check.

The best way to enjoy the smells and scents of essential oils is with help of diffusers. Easily available in the market, these diffusers are the best way to use essential oils and use them to make your home smell beautiful. As the winter season is fast approaching, there are many people who suffer from seasonal colds, wheezing and asthma that gets bad during the cold weather.

A diffuser is part humidifier, part air purifier and it helps to enjoy the aroma of essential oils the best way. All you have to do is put in some drops of essential oil along with a small amount of water. The ultrasonic technology in the diffuser will break the mixture of essential oil and water in millions of microparticles and disperses them into air, getting rid of odors and creates a relaxing atmosphere, giving you a wonderful therapeutic treatment with the oil being used.

As the holiday season is fast approaching, it is time to fill your home with the right scents that help you create a wonderful and warm environment inside, leaving behind the cold and gloom outside. There is a variety of essential oils that can help you feel good and warm with their natural and therapeutic effects.

This chapter brings some of the top holiday winter warming blends for diffusers that will help you enjoy the festivities and be happy.

1. *Spiced cedar blend for winters*

This winter blend is a great way to make your holidays nice smelling and cheerful even if you do not have the apple scented essential oil. This recipe gives you the idea of how you can add that spicy aroma to your blend by adding just a hint of sweet orange oil. The scent in sweet orange is enough to give the illusion of apples without making the blend too citrusy.

All you will need to make spiced cedar blend is:

- 2 drops of Sweet Orange

- 6 drops Ginger extract

- 4 drops Cinnamon Bark

Mix these three ingredients together and you have the perfect spiced cedar blend ready for the winter holidays that you can enjoy in days to come.

2. *Gingerbread cookie blend*

Even if you are out of allspices but want to add that special aroma to your environment, this is the perfect recipe. All you need to use is drop of black pepper and you will get that traditional spicy gingerbread aroma. If you want, you can use nutmeg instead of allspice to give your blend a sweeter and slighter fragrance.

All you need for this blend is:

- 2 drops of Cassia

- 6 drops of Ginger

- 2 drops of Clove

- 2 drops of Allspice

Mix them all together and use in a diffuser with a little water for the effect gingerbread cookie aroma, just right for this holiday season.

3. *Candy cane blend*

Candy Cane is a sugary sweet treat for everyone and takes you back in the days of childhood. If you do not have Cassia, the essential ingredient for candy cane, you can use Cinnamon bark in its place. However you should know that Cassia gives the blend a more candy-like aroma that is closer to the original thing.

For this blend you will need:

- 2 drops Spearmint

- 2 drops Cassia

- 6 drops Peppermint

Blend them all together and use them in your diffuser for the sweet candy cane aroma in this holiday season.

4. *Holiday cheer blend*

This is a nice, warm and rich smelling blend that is fit for winter season. However, you must know that the quality of ginger depends on how strong or light you want it. Try it out with two drops first and if you want to add some more, you can do that later after checking how it smells. Experiment and you will know what it is all about.

All you require for this particular blend is:

- 4 drops of Sweet Orange

- 4 drops of Ginger

- 2 drops of Cinnamon Bark

- 2 drops of Pine

Mix them all together and use them in this coming season for a really cheerful effect around the house.

5. *Long winter pleasant blend*

This particular blend gives off a very nice aroma that reminds you of pine trees and combined with cedar wood, it gives off an earthy whiff that is neither to subtle or over-powering and makes a great choice for holiday season. All the ingredients blend really nicely with other two oils and make it a crisp and refreshing aroma.

To make this blend you need:

- 4 drops of Fir Needle

- 2 drop of Cedarwood

- 2 – 4 drops of Frankincense

- 2 drop of Rosemary

Combine all these ingredients together and you will get a perfect blend for entertaining guests.

6. *Frosty boughs*

This is an absolutely refreshing and energizing combination of mint oils and gives you a chance to freshen up your surroundings. If you want a mintier aroma, you need to lessen the quantity of fir needle. If you like the pine scent more, try to use one portion of spearmint with two portions of fir needles and it will work out perfect.

Here is what you will need to make this blend:

- 2 drop of Peppermint

- 4drops of Spearmint

- 2 drop of Cedar wood

- 4 drop of Fir Needle

Mix them together and you will have a perfect frost boughs aroma ready to scent your surroundings.

7. *Christmas tree*

This blend is a combination of patchouli with fir needle that is earthier and less woody and you will feel as if you are standing in a green forest and actually enjoying the fresh smells.

For this blend you need:

- 3 – 4 drops of Fir Needle

- 2 drops of Patchouli

- 2 – 4 drops of Pine

Check out the type of patchouli you have as you might need to increase the quantity of fir needle to balance the blend if needed.

8. *Wild fall blend*

This is a unique blend that will keep your house smelling fresh and build immunity in the cold winter days.

All you need for this blend:

- 4 drops of Wild Orange

- 4 drops of Patchouli

- 2 drop of Clove

Mix all these oils together and you will be ready for winters.

9. *Autumn leaves blend*

To make your home smell like fresh autumn leaves and enjoy the season, go for this blend.

All you need for this blend:

- 6 drops of Wild Orange

- 2 drop of Rosemary

- 2 drop of Ginger

Mix them all together and put in the diffuser and you will just love this blend.

All these winter blends are unique and help you create a perfect setting for the cold days when you want to inhale those fresh and earthy smell and imagine yourself a part of them. These holiday diffuser blends for winter will help you enjoy this time and make it memorable with your family and friends. Try them out and you will feel different.

Chapter 02: Calming Essential Oil Blends for Winter

With winters comes stress and tensions that have partly to do with the weather and partly due to the inability to go out and refresh your senses. However, there is nothing to worry about as essential oils play a very key role in calming the senses and giving a therapeutic effect to the mind.

Scents have a very powerful effect on our emotions and moods and we can use some of the most heavenly smelling volatile oils that contain aromatic molecules to cross the blood and brain barrier. Their direct effect on our brain helps to ease stress, anxiety, fear and depression and make us feel better. While it is significant to know that severe cases of depression and anxiety cannot be cured with these essential oils, yet they can help you reduce these problems and with help of medical care you can help to relax and feel better.

There is a huge variety of essential oils that are easily available in the market hat help you alleviate the symptoms of stress and anxiety and help you remain calm and tranquil even in the worst of situations when you are cooped inside and cannot go out due to severe weather conditions.

They can be used all day long without any fear or running out as only a few drops are used and mixed with water, they give off heavily aromas for a long time when used in a diffuser. With their clean and healthy scents, essential oils are a great way to get rid of symptoms of depression, anxiety and mood swings that often hit us badly. The uplifting power of essential oils helps us remain calm and focus on our activities in a positive way.

This chapter discuses some of the calming essential oil blends for winters so that you can benefit from this great natural resource during the winter months and enjoy aromatherapy at home.

10.Allergy Relief

This is a great blend that helps to get rid of all types of allergies particularly those associated with cold weather.

For this blend you require:

- 2 drops of Peppermint

- 2 drops of Lavender

- 2 drops of Lemon

Put them all together and use them in the diffuser and see how well it controls your allergy this season.

11. Calming effect blend

This blend is best for settling down at night and relaxing. It can be used before bedtime as it also helps to keep the kids calm and putting them to sleep becomes easy when they are hyperactive and do not want to give up play.

Here is what you need for this blend:

- *4* drops Lavender

- 4drops Wild Orange

- 4 drops Roman Chamomile

Just mix them all together and put them in a diffuser and see how it calms down the children and puts them to sleep so that you can also follow them to bed and enjoy a good night's sleep.

12. *Breathe easy*

This blend is simply marvelous because it keeps your respiratory function working just right and helps to clear off the congestion during the cold seasons. It protects you from the chest and throat infections that are rampant during the cold weather.

For this blend you need:

- 4 drops Lemon

- 2 drop Lime

- 4 drops Peppermint

- 2drop Rosemary

- 4 drops Eucalyptus

- 2 drop Clove

All these ingredients are really good and contain therapeutic properties that keep your allergies and ailments at bay and protect you against all seasonal problems that come with the cold. Just mix them all together and see how they work.

13. *Headache reliever blend*

White peppermint is known for alleviating headaches when it is rubbed on the temples and back of the neck and clary sage is known to help for aches during hormonal imbalance. These two are known to provide relief even to the toughest of headaches.

To make this blend you need:

- 2 drops of Marjoram
- 2 drops of Thyme
- 2 drops of Rosemary
- 2 drops of Peppermint
- 2 drops of Lavender

Mix all these essential oils together and use in a diffuser to relief all types of headaches that plague you during winter season.

14. *Winding down blend*

This is the best way to cool down after a long and hectic day and when you feel all hyped up and unable to relax. Just use this blend and see how it helps to relieve stress.

All you require to make this blend:

- 8 drops of Lavender

- 4 drops of Cedar wood

- 4 drops of Wild Orange

- 2 drops of Ylang Ylang

Mix these essential oils together and use them in a diffuser and see how they help you deal more rationally with things and how calm and serene you feel.

15. Ginger stress relief blend

This is a great blend as it helps to reduce the feelings of anxiety and uplifts the moods by encouraging circulation and digestion.

What you need for this blend:

- 4 drops of Frankincense

- 3 drops of Ginger

- 5 drops of Orange

- 4 drops of Cedar wood

Mix all these oils together and you will get a perfect ginger stress relief blend that will help you enjoy better quality of life.

Chapter 03: Warm and Aromatic Essential Oil Blends

As the winter season approaches, it is time for cozy sweaters and oversized socks along with hot beverages that help to fight cold and stay warm. You can make your cold winter days and nights perfect by warming up your living areas with comforting and seasonal essential oil blends.

Not only these blends give a feeling or warmth but they smell heavenly too and in their purest form, they help you feel good. Whether you are feeling down or you have a headache, the right choice of an essential oil will get you moving and active within no time. All you need is to make the right selection so that you get a blend that is perfect for you and brightens up your area with sweet scents.

You can use these oil blends in a diffuser but if you want to get some added warmth, you can also use a censer and it will give you that warm and toasty smell when the oil burns. This chapter discuses some of the best oil blends that are warm and aromatic and help you enjoy this season.

16. Sugar and spice blend

This is one particular blend that is well liked by many people due to its sweet yet spicy effect. A combination of citrus and spice, it creates a very warm and welcoming environment. Clove oil is particular knowns for giving way to feelings of love and acceptance which is perfect for holiday seasons especially Christmas.

For this blend you require:

- 2 drops of Sweet Orange

- 2 drops of Bergamot

- 1 drops of Clove

- 1 drops of Cinnamon

Mix all these essential oils and you will find your home all cozy and inviting, ready for the holiday season.

17. *Winter Wonderland blend*

The woody and earthy scent of cedar wood and pine is a stress reliever that will help you sit back and relax and enjoy time with family when everyone is in frenzy around you to complete all their shopping well before time.

All you need for this blend:

- 2 drops Pine

- 2 drops Cedar wood

- 1 drops Orange

- 1 drops Nutmeg

Mix these varieties of essential oils together and you will enjoy this blend greatly for giving a warm and inviting scent to your home that will keep everyone relaxed and calk.

18. Immunity boosting blend

As the name goes, this blend is made with naturally antiseptic essential oils that will help to boost your immune system and keep it working it perfect order. During the holiday seasons, cold and flu are rampant and using these oils will help your immune system stay strong and ready to fight the cold. Eucalyptus and pine are known for clearing the respiratory system and they give a warm feeling that leads to better health in the long run.

Here is what you need to make this blend:

- 2 drops of Eucalyptus
- 2 drops of Lavender
- 1 drops of Thyme
- 1 drops of Pine

Combine all these oils together and you will get a perfect blend that will not only boost your immunity but also keep you warm, ready to face the upcoming holidays and enjoy yourself.

19. Warm Chai blend

If you love a hot cup of tea or chai as it is known in India, then you will definitely love this essential oil blend as it is just right for filling your house with warmth and fun.

Make your holiday seasons more toasty and cheerful with the warm chai blend that will become your favorite.

What you need to make this blend:

- 4 drops Cardamom

- 3 drops Cinnamon

- 1 drop Clove

- 1 drop Nutmeg

- 3 drops Ginger

Mix these essential oils together and you will be surprised at eh feeling or warmth and happiness it generates. Use it in diffuser or even in a censer and you will love it.

20. *Winter Sunrise blend*

Winter brings colds, blocked sinuses and other problems and there is no other way to deal with them than with natural products. These sweet smelling essential oils are the key to getting rid of these common ailments like cold and flu and they keep you al warm and healthy for the holidays. Aromatherapy is fast becoming one of the best way to treat problems like cold and flu that do not require medicines or treatments.

What you need for this blend:

- 4 drops Sweet Orange

- 4 drops Rosemary

- 4 drops Ginger

- 4 drops Eucalyptus

- 2 drop Cinnamon

- 2 drop Clove

Mix these essential oils together and use them in a diffuser and you will see the difference very soon. With their aroma, they will help you fight these problems and give the natural winter sunrise effect.

21. *Healthy Orange Blend*

This blend not only smells great but it is also very good for health as it contains clove and rosemary, the essential ingredients for so many medicines.

For this blend you need:

- 4 drops of Wild Orange

- 3 drops of Clove

- 3 drops of Rosemary

Put them all together in a diffuser and see the magic.

There is a variety of warm and aromatic essential oil blends that can be used in diffusers to create a perfectly warm and welcoming environment in your home. All you need to do is find the best combination that works for you so that you can enjoy better health and environment.

Chapter 04: Warm EO Blends to Reduce Stress and Tension

When it comes to reducing stress and tension and living a better quality life, warm essential oil blends are a great choice. It is because derived from the plants, fruits and other sources, these are the purest scenes that contain the properties of their source and help to alleviate several ailments.

Stress and tension is very common in society these days and people from all sections of life experience them at one point or another. Taking medicines and popping tablets on regular basis is not the way to deal with them as they have serious side effects and they are addictive too. Essential oils are being used by people since early times when there were no other ways of treatment. History tells us that various cultures have been using aromatherapy to treat patients that includes china, India, Egypt and southern Europe.

The best thing about using these essential oils is that they are the most natural form of oil that is extracted from flowers, leaves, barks or roots of plants and they provide a much needed relief from problems like stress and anxiety. This chapter discusses the benefits of warm essential oil blends that can help to reduce tension and stress and create a feeling or love and peace in your house. If used the right way and in the right quantity, these essential oils can do wonders for people who suffer from feelings of stress and want to get rid of them without resorting to medication.

22.Lavender Blend

It is one of the most commonly used essential oil due to its benefits. It has a calming and relaxing effect that is also good for restoring nervous system and inner peace. It helps in better sleeping patterns and help to cure problems like restlessness, feelings of irritation, panic attacks and general feelings of anxiety.

A number of patients suffering from tension and stress were tested with lavender and it was found that when used in diffuser, lavender has anxiolytic effects that means it acts as a tranquilizer that can be used to relieve anxiety and reduce tension and irritability. A few drops of lavender essential oil in a diffuser during the day can keep your home environment really calm and help you get rid of all tensions and stress without taking any medication.

23.Bergamot

It has a distinctive floral taste and smell and it is most often found in earl grey tea. It has a calming effort and it is used to treat depression by providing positive energy and also helps insomnia patients by inducing relaxation and reducing agitation.

Research has shown that when this blended essential oil was used in diffusers, it helped in treating depression among patients. A combination of lavender and bergamot essential oil is very effective for a stress free environment.

24.Chamomile

Chamomile has a very peaceful and calming scent and it helps in inner harmony and reduces feelings of irritability, overthinking as well as anxiety and stress. During a research on effects of chamomile it was discovered that it contains the right antidepressant that can help in calming the brain and gives a feeling of inner peace.

Chamomile is the most commonly used essential oil and most of the people like to use it in soaps for better effects. Chamomile essential oil can be used in a diffuser for a perfectly harmonious home environment.

25.Frankincense

This is a great essential oil that helps to treat depression and anxiety as it provides calming and tranquil energy along with spiritual grounding. When used in aromatherapy, it helps in meditation as it relaxes the mind.

When mixed with bergamot and lavender oils in equal proportion, it also has a very positive effect on various pains and aches.

26.Ylang Ylang

It is a popular essential oil that is frequently used in treatment of depression and anxiety as it contains calming and uplifting properties. It helps to induce a cheerful mood and gives way to feelings of optimism and fearfulness. It has also been found very beneficial in calming agitation as well as nervous palpitation and also helps as a sedative to patients who suffer from stress and tension.

All these warm blends of essential oils are very effective for reducing stress and tension and they also make sure that you feel happy and cheerful after using them with their heavenly smells and therapeutic effects.

Chapter 05: Cozy Winter Warming Blends for Diffusers

Winters are time of hot beverages and cozy clothes and if you want some fresh and natural smells in your house, there is nothing better than essential oils to warm your soul and keep you all toasty. These lovely smells take you back to your childhood and help to remember those wonderful days.

You can stay away from the cold and enjoy the fresh scents while staying healthy at the same time with some of the best essential oils.

27. Cozy Holiday Blend

This cozy holiday blend help you keep your home fresh and the inside environment crisp.

Here is what you need to make this blend:

- 1 drop of Wild Orange

- 1 drop of Cassia

- 1 drop of White Fir

Mix them all together and you will have heavenly smelling blend that will make your home feel cozy and comfortable.

28.Apple Pie Blend

You can make this blend to make your house fresh with the smell of apple pie without actually making any or without using any applesauce.

What you need for this blend:

- 3 drops of Clove

- 3 drops of Cinnamon

- 3 drops of Ginger

Mix them together and you will enjoy fresh scent that is also very good for immunity and better health.

29.Minty Fresh blend

This blend is the best for winter season when you want some fresh and citrusy smells to make the inside environment crisp and healthy.

What you require for this blend:

- 6 drops Spearmint

- 3 drops Lemon

- 2 drop Lavender

- 2 drop Eucalyptus

- 2 drop Cedar wood

You will have a clean and clear house after using this essential oil blend that will battle stagnant and musty air and get rid of all mental and physical fatigue.

30.Rose and black pepper blend

This is a great combination as it helps greatly in keeping the room cozy and also works wonders when used for massage as it helps to stimulate blood circulation and encourages feelings of love and warmth.

What you need for this blend:

- 4 drops Black pepper

- 3 drops Patchouli

- 2 drop Rose

- 4 drops Cardamom

Add all these essential oils together and enjoy a cozy and fresh smell in your house.

31.Rosemary and Lavender Blend

This is a great blend for immunity as lavender is known for its therapeutic powers and when combined with rosemary it helps blood circulation and reduces inflammation, giving feelings of good health.

What you need for this blend:

- 4 drops Rosemary

- 4 drops Juniper

- 8 drops Ravensara

- 8 drops Lavender

Mix all these essential oils together and you will get a great aromatic blend that will help you built immunity and live well.

32.Oatmeal Cookies Blend

If you love oatmeal cookies and their smell when it permeates the house, this is the one for you.

What you need for this blend:

- 3 drops of Cedar wood

- 3 drops of Cassia

- 3 drops of Wild Orange

Blend them all together and use in a diffuser for sweet and irresistible scents.

33. *Winter cabin blend*

If you wish you were at some cabin enjoying the outdoors, this blend will give you exactly this.

For this blend you need:

- 4 drops of Fir needle

- 4 drops of Cedar wood

- 4 drops of Wild Orange

Mix them together and make your holidays more exciting

34. *Forest Blend*

If you want your house to smell as fresh as a forest with hint of grass, flowers and clean air, this is the right blend.

For this blend you need:

- 4 drops of Lime

- 4 drops of Lemon

- 2 drop of Wild Orange

- 2 drop of Bergamot

- 2 drop of White Fir

Mix them all and you will just love the result.

35.Fire warmth Blend

If you want to get the warmth and the coziness that fire brings, then this blend is a perfect choice.

For this blend you need:

- 4 drops of Cinnamon

- 3 drops of Clove

- 3 drops of White Fir

Mix them together and you will just enjoy the feeling of warmth and coziness it inspires.

Conclusion

Ever since their therapeutic and health properties have become common, essential oils have become an important part of our lives sometimes scenting our homes and sometimes helping us stay healthy by strengthening our immune system. Whether you are looking for a way to manage your ailments and problems or seek spiritual enlightening, these small drops of oil can do wonders. This ebook explores the benefits of using essential oil for your health and brings the top 35 winter warming blends for diffusers that you can use for various health and cleaning purposes.

More and more people are running to the benefits of essential oils to fight the cold and flu as well as stress and anxiety that is becoming very common in our lives. As the winter season approaches, using essential oil blends is the best thing to do when it comes to maintaining a fresh and crisp environment in your home and fighting common ailments that strike in this season.

This ebook provides the right information that will help you understand how you can use these natural sources to fight winter and remain warm with some of the most heavenly smelling essential oil blends right in your home.

Thank you for downloading and reading our ebook as it has been specifically written to help you live a better quality life, build immunity and keep away from common ailments and aches without using any medicines. You just need to understand the therapeutic benefits of essential oils and how they can be used with diffusers for best results.

If you have any questions regarding our ebook, you can contact us and we will be happy to answer them for you. Happy Reading!

FREE Bonus Reminder

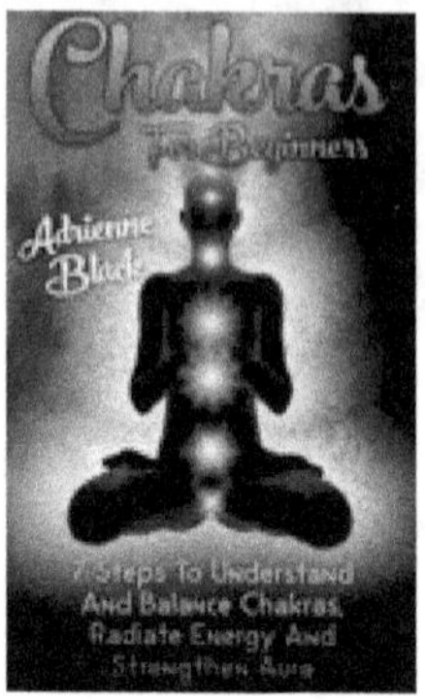

If you have not grabbed it yet, please go ahead and download your special bonus E book *"Chakras for Beginners. 7 Steps To Understand And Balance Chakras, Radiate Energy, And Strengthen Aura"*.

Simply Click the Button Below

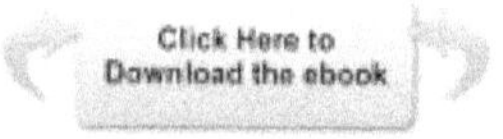

OR Go to This Page

http://lifehacksworld.com/free

BONUS #2: More Free & Discounted Books & Products

Do you want to receive more Free/Discounted Books or Products?

We have a mailing list where we send out our new Books or Products when they go free or with a discount on Amazon. Click on the link below to sign up for Free & Discount Book & Product Promotions.

=> Sign Up for Free & Discount Book & Product Promotions <=

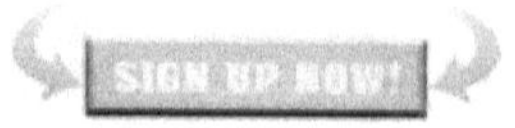

OR Go to this URL

http://zbit.ly/1WBb1Ek